Namasté

I want to thank the teachers and students I have had over the years and who have made my journey with yoga so interesting. Thank you for all the inspiration you have given me and for making this book possible. The yoga masters who no longer live among us, live on with every new person who immerses themselves in the yoga tradition.

Sri Swami Sivananda, Sri Swami Satyananda, Sri Tirumalai Krishnamacharya, Sri Swami Vishnudevananda, Sri K. Pattabhi Jois, Osho, Swami Nirdosha, Swami Omananda, Swami Janakananda, Ole Schmidt, Turiya, Maryam Abrishami and Sanna Kuittinen.

Everyone who has searched for answers to what they perceived through an activated ajna chakra. In yoga, they have learned the principles behind the universe, the collective consciousness, and the creative power, Kundalini Shakti. The duality behind everything, both what we see and what we do not see. Together we help to pass on the previous secret knowledge, about our gunas, nadis, and chakras, to anyone who wants to be seen.

THE AUTHOR

Shreyananda Natha is the author of over twelve titles on yoga. Among other things, he has written the most comprehensive books on yoga in Swedish – Everything About Yoga and the study book The Yoga Bible. He is also a certified yoga and meditation teacher according to EYTF's international guidelines and has undergone a multi-year yoga teacher training under the leadership of Swami Omananda at Satyananda Ashram. Shreyananda Natha holds the highest initiation in the Tantric Natha Order. He travels frequently to Asia and India to improve himself, and to gain knowledge and inspiration. He has immersed himself in the tantric rituals and is known for his extensive knowledge of yoga, deep relaxation, and meditation

There is no authority that can say what yoga is. When you give yourself fully and completely, and experience yoga without limitations or doubts, when you become one with the true experience in yourself, the real encounter with yoga arises. Only then do you understand what yoga is – for you. You are no longer limited by ornament, shyness and artificial thought patterns that lie as a filter between you and the transformation. Yoga is a cultural-historical wealth that is still passed on from teacher to student and helps man to find his way back to his true nature. It opens us up and attracts awareness.

ESOTERIC
YOGA

The path of the right and left hands!

Cover & Graphic Design

Mattias Långström

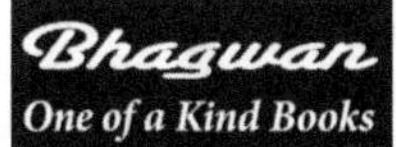

ESOTERIC YOGA

The path of the right and left hands!

ISBN 9789198735826

✺✸✺

It strengthens our self-esteem, and our entire person's spectrum of possibilities suddenly becomes visible to us. Yoga is not difficult. You do not have to be vegan or able to stand on your head. You just need to practice your yoga regularly and the rest will come by itself.

With all the love from the universe – Aum Shanti Shreyananda Natha.

ESOTERIC YOGA

THE WAY OF HIDDEN KNOWLEDGE

Esoteric means "inaccessible" or "only for the initiated", and is most often used to denote the hidden wisdom or secret spiritual knowledge that underlies philosophical systems. The term esoteric can also refer to the teachings and practices of supersensible experiences that require special preparation and training, often under the guidance of an experienced teacher.

Why is knowledge hidden, one might wonder? The answer is multifaceted, but in addition to the fact that the mysterious and hidden have an appeal to new students, it has a purely practical explanation. For example, if someone is only temporarily curious, they will most likely forget a mantra told to them, even if the mantra could be life saving. Tradition - the knowledge of it - will go nowhere. If, on the other hand, a person were to undergo demanding yogic and tantric training for years, that person will be more likely to remember the mantra. By keeping the knowledge hidden, it ensures that the knowledge is passed on and preserved for the future.

According to an old prophecy, the hidden, esoteric, tantric acts would one day be practiced quite openly - during Kali's age - which is now. It allows me to write about the most advanced tantric rituals that have previously been hidden. However, I can not reveal everything. I can not tell you everything about things that can be abused. For example, I will not reveal the most powerful mantra there is, the shodasi mantra. A mantra that can replace all other secret mantras and gives the holder the power to influence everything in the macro and microcosm: the power of life and death; success and defeat. However, I can tell you about other previously hidden ones, the rituals that are refined through training and that give the adept an increased awareness and increased vitality to deal with everything in life successfully. There is no point in not telling about that knowledge, in not passing it on. It would be like not telling interested people where they can find the best running shoes. Everything that can make it easier for people to have increased vitality and joy of life must now be acknowledged. The time has come. The time is now. The time is yours. Good luck!

THE PATH OF THE RIGHT AND LEFT HANDS
In tantra – which is the basis of all yoga, the hidden knowledge is preserved in two different directions, or paths.

We talk about the path of the right hand (dakshinachara), and the path of the left hand (vamachara).

Both paths aim to awaken Kundalini shakti and give the practitioner cosmic power. The difference is that instead of striving to become one with the divine as in dakshinachara, in vamachara tantra one strives to become divine. However, both paths are considered equal ways of enlightening the Indian tantric practitioners, although vamachara is considered the faster and more dangerous way.

DAKSHINACHARA

Dakshinachara is also described as the inner way, or the path of inner meditation. Rituals are based on the practitioner's own interior, such as Kriya yoga.

VAMACHARA

Vamachara, the path of external meditation, is often the path that people know in tantra, is where the adept gets help from things and experiences in the outside world to expand power. For example, the use of meat and wine in the maithuna ritual (tantric intercourse).

Both paths use secret mantras and yantras in their tantric rituals to achieve their purposes.

MANTRA SHASTRA

Mantra shastra is the foundation of all spiritual practice and has a central role in all esoteric yoga.

MANTRA

The most basic mantra is Aum, also known as the pranava mantra, the source of all mantras.

Two types of mantras which have a literal meaning are:

1.) SAGUNA MANTRA

Mantras that represent and invoke a deity, god or goddess for spiritual self-realization. Saguna mantras create visual patterns through repeated chanting until the deity appears in true form.

Some examples of saguna mantras are:

a) Om Namah Shivaya. Greetings to Shiva.
b) Om Nam Narayanaya. Greeting to God over harmony and balance.
c) Gayatri mantra. Dedicated to the goddess Gayatri.
d) Mahamrityunjaya mantra. Dedicated to Shiva.

More similar mantras are shanti mantra, Ram, Sita, Om Aing Saraswati Namaha, etc.

2.) NIRGUNA MANTRA

Mantras that are formless, abstract and represent the universe as a whole and not in any specific form are called nirguna mantras. These mantras require a higher form of concentration as they do not refer to any actual form. They are for deeper meditation and with regular practice, siddhis (paranormal abilities) are obtained.

The use of nirguna mantras is primarily to become one with the absolute or to identify with the divine in the universe.

Some examples of nirguna mantras are:

a) Om (Aum).
Om is the original mantra, the root of all sounds and letters that create language and thoughts.
b) So Ham.

We unconsciously utter this mantra every time we breathe. On inhalation - So, and on exhalation - Ham. So Ham means - I am that, beyond the limitations of the mind and body, I am one with the infinite. I am. That's me.

There are primarily ten different types of mantras without a literal meaning:

1. Shanti (siddhi) mantra – to free oneself from disease, fear, imagination and other problems.
2. Stambhan mantra – to make living beings unable to move.

3. Mohana mantra – used to create attraction.

4. Uchchatan mantra – used to create mental imbalance in people.

5. Vashikaran mantra – used to turn someone into a slave.

6. Akarshan mantra – used to acquire wealth and material happiness.

7. Jrambhan mantra – used to change human behavior.

8. Vidweshan mantra – used to make two people enemies.

9. Maran mantra – used to kill someone.

10. Paustik mantra – used to become a successful person on all levels.

SRI VIDYA MANTRA – SHODASI MANTRA

Sri yantra – also known as Sri Chakra- is called the mother of all yantras because all other yantras are descended from it. It is the most powerful yantra and symbolizes the creation of the cosmos and all life. Sri Vidya is worshiped by the tantrics of both the right and left hands.

SRI YANTRA

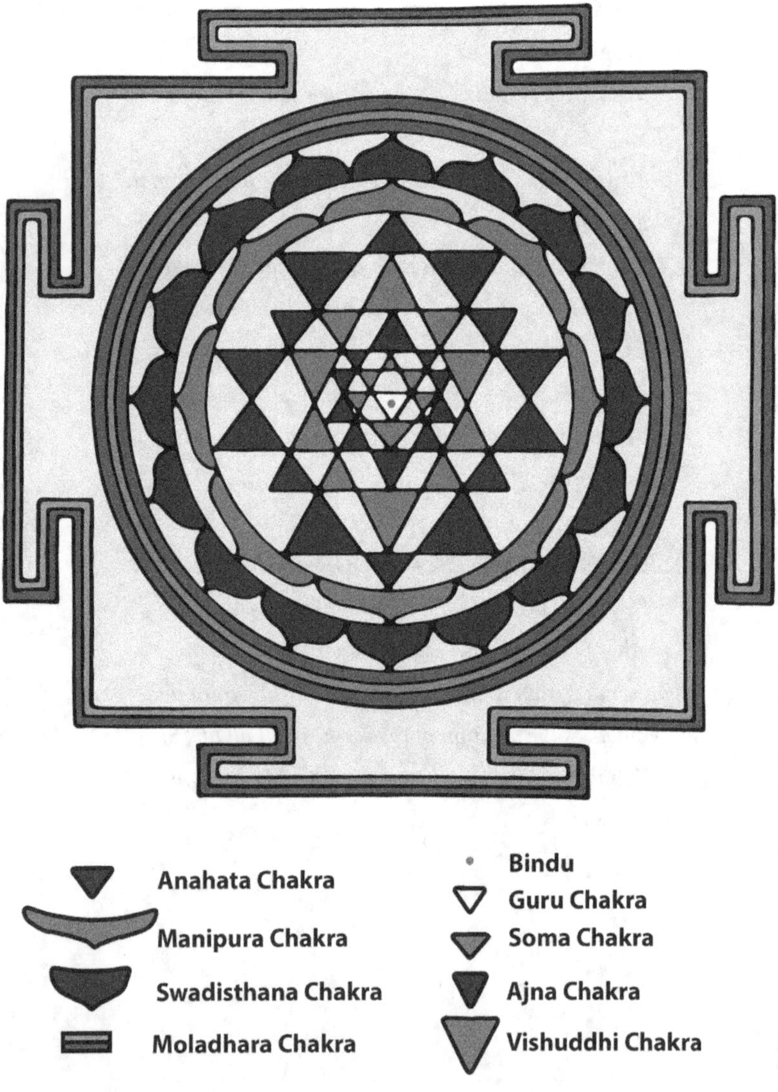

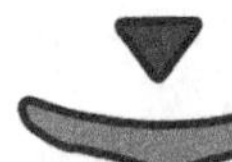
Anahata Chakra

Manipura Chakra

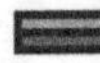
Swadisthana Chakra

Moladhara Chakra

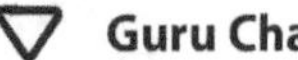
Bindu

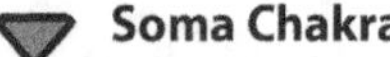
Guru Chakra

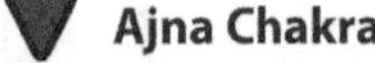
Soma Chakra

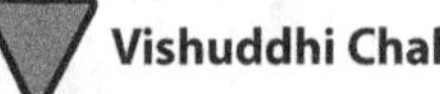
Ajna Chakra

Vishuddhi Chakra

Sri Vidya or Sri Chakra represents Sri Lalita or Tripura Sundari – Shakti in her most beautiful form, a sixteen year old beauty. Sri Lalita is represented by sixteen syllables as she is also associated with sixteen desires.

Since Sri yantra is the most powerful yantra, it also possesses the most powerful mantra – the shodasi mantra. It is quite logical if you think about it, as each form also has a sound.

The shodasi mantra is the most secret and protected mantra there is and is completely impossible to find out about – unless you are initiated by a guru. Forget all the pages on the internet that claim to know the mantra because it is completely wrong and unreasonable. If you have undergone all the trials that it means to be initiated, you just do not give it away – especially not on the internet.

Normally, one does not initiate the shodasi mantra directly; it is the guru who decides which time and place is most favorable. Generally, you are first initiated in the bala mantra, then depending on your maturity and insight, you are initiated in the panchadasi mantra. The panchadasi mantra is a mantra made up of fifteen stages syllables. If the guru then thinks that the adept is ready for final liberation, he is initiated into the shodasi

*mantra and gains knowledge of the secret sixteenth
stage.*

*In order for the adept to achieve complete liberation
and obtain magical abilities, so-called siddhis, he must
recite the mantra nine hundred thousand times and add
purascharana each time at the end.*

BRAHMA VIDYA – THE BIGGEST SECRET

*Shodashi vidya is also referred to as Brahma vidya:
Brahman (the world soul) and Vidya (the knowledge).
Brahman is rendered into mantra form in shodasi vidya
and because of this, it is guarded as the greatest secret.*

*If the practitioner has the opportunity to reach the
fourth level of consciousness, known as turiya(super-
consciousness), then it is most likely he is also prepared
to go beyond this, to reach the fifth level of consciousness
known as turiyatita. Turiyatita can be reached without
difficulty when the shodasi mantra is recited regularly.*

*Therefore, by reaching turiyatita (the fifth level of
consciousness) and by reciting the shodasi mantra, you
become one with Brahman. There is nothing after this.*

*What happens when a person is transformed into turiy-
atita? The soul is replaced by the world soul, the divine*

consciousness. You become divine and gain divine power.

This is also something that can be experienced in a moment of near death, a person is never the same after such an experience.

BIJA MANTRA

Mantras often used in tantra are bija mantras. They are different sounds that have no direct literal meaning, but that have the power to create a great transformation and expansion of the physical, emotional and mental forces. They are called bees or seed mantra, or so-called-magical sounds.

The approximately fifty sacred sounds from the Sanskrit alphabet (bija mantras) are primarily resonants for the seven major chakras. Properly stated, they activate the energy in different chakras and purify and balance the mind and body. They also increase the power of various mantra compositions.

AIM

After Om (Aum) the second most common bija mantra is Aim, pronounced – Aym. Aim is the feminine aspect of Om and often follows Om in various mantras. Om and Aim consist of two compound vowels and therefore include all sounds. A + u creates Om and A + i creates Aim.

Om helps to purify the mental and Aim helps to focus in different ways.

Just as Om is the sound of the invisible, Aim is the sound of the visible. Om is the sound of the unmanifested and Aim is the sound of the manifested. The principle of consciousness and energy. Shiva and Shakti. Therefore, one can often hear Aim in Shakti mantras. Mantras of the Divine Mother.

Aim is the bija mantra for Saraswati, the goddess of knowledge and speech. Aim helps us in education, art, expression, communication and is good for all forms of school work in general. Aim is also a guru mantra and helps us to have greater knowledge in everything. It also helps us with concentration during the recitation of the mantras.

HRIM

After Om and Aim, Hrim, pronounced "Hreem", is the most common bija mantra.

It is a combination of the sound Ha, which stands for energy/prana, space and light with the sound of Ra, which stands for fire, light and learning; and the sound A, which stands for energy, concentration and motivation.

Hrim is bija mantra for Shakti or Parvati.

Hrim is a mantra for magic, attraction, love and power. It brings us joy, ecstasy, passion, and complete happiness.

Hrim is a specific mantra for the heart (hridaya in Sanskrit) on all its different levels: spiritually, emotionally, as a chakra, and as a physical organ.

SRIM

Srim, pronounced "Shreem", is one of the most common bija mantras due to its positive properties. It attracts everything that is good, favorable and helps us develop in a positive way.

Srim is the bija mantra of Lakshmi, and is also called the Ramas bija, when used for the worship of Lord Rama.

Srim is the mantra of faith, devotion, refuge and surrender. It can be used to take refuge in or indulge in various deities and obtain their favors.

Srim relates to the heart more from a feminine and sentimental perspective, while Hrim relates to the heart from a masculine, pranic or functional perspective.

Srim is often used with Hrim asHrim relates to the sun and Srim relates to the moon.

KRIM

Krim is pronounced "Kreem", and is the most important bija mantra that begins with a harsh consonant. Krim begins with Ka, the first consonant in Sanskrit and which shows manifested prana and the initial phase of energy. To Ka it adds the Ra sound – the sound of fire and the A sound that concentrates power like the other Shakti mantras. Krim creates light just like Hrim and Srim but on a more specific and actualized level.

Krim is the bija mantra of Kali, the goddess of time, destruction and transformation. Kali also creates the highest energy level within us.

Krim is the mantra of work, yoga and the energy of transformation. It is known to be a bija mantra for yoga practitioners andis applied to awaken Kundalini shakti within us. Krim stimulates higher perceptiveness and higher prana and works to stabilize pratyahara within us. The mantra can create contact with any deity.

KLIM

*Klim is pronounced "Kleem" and is the softer, more fe-
minine aspect of Krim. Just as Krim is electric, Klim has
a magnetic quality and attracts things to us.*

*Klim relates to akarshana shakti or the law of attrac-
tion.*

*Klim is the bija mantra for Krishna and Sundari, the
goddesses of love and beauty. It is also the bija mantra
over all desires (kama bija) and helps us achieve our
inner desires in life. Klim is the mantra of love and devotion and increases the level of love within us. Because
of this, it is one of the most used mantras.*

STRIM

*Strim, pronounced "Streem", is composed of the Sa
sound which stands for stability and the Ta sound which
creates expansion, with the A sound which provides us
with energy, direction and motivation.*

*Strim is known to be the peace mantra, the so-called
shanti bija. The mantra Strim provides the power to
have children, to enrich something nutritionally, to pro-
tect and to guide. It is similar to Srim but stronger and
has a more stabilizing effect.*

Strim is the bija mantra of the Hindu goddess Tara (not the Buddhist Tara). Hindu Tara is associated with Durga, often called Durga-Tara, a guarding and protective form of the goddess.

HUM

Hum is pronounced "Hoom", and is one of the most important bija mantras along with Om, Aim and Hrim. It is said to be pranava, the sound of Lord Shiva.

Hum is the great agni or fire mantra, and can increase the fire within us at all different levels. Everything from the fire of consciousness, the pranic fire, and to the burning of the body.

Hum is also a weapon, a protecting mantra that can be used to destroy negativity with its enlightening fire. It is also called the bija mantra of anger (krodha bija).

Hum relates to a violent form of the goddess, like Kali, Chandi or Chinnamasta.

Hum is especially used to raise Kundalini shakti in combination with breathing and with concentration on the navel (Manipura chakra).

SECRET CHAKRAS

In yoga, people usually talk about seven or eight larger chakras that are located along the spine and at the top of the head. If you count Bindu visarga as a chakra, then you say that there are eight major important chakras in a human being. Bindu is located on the top of the back of the head and, according to popular belief, has no kshetram.

In the hidden tradition you get to learn a big secret: that Bindu's placement on the back of the head is actually the chakra's kshetram. That Bindu is located above the Sahasrara chakra and is called Sunya. When the Kundalini shakti reaches the Sunya – the black chakra, one is transformed into a deity and receives divine qualities.

In addition to Sunya, there are other chakras that are hidden: Guru, Nirvana, Indu, Manas and Tala (Lalana) chakras are placed in the head and Hrit chakra is placed just below the Anahata chakra, the heart chakra.

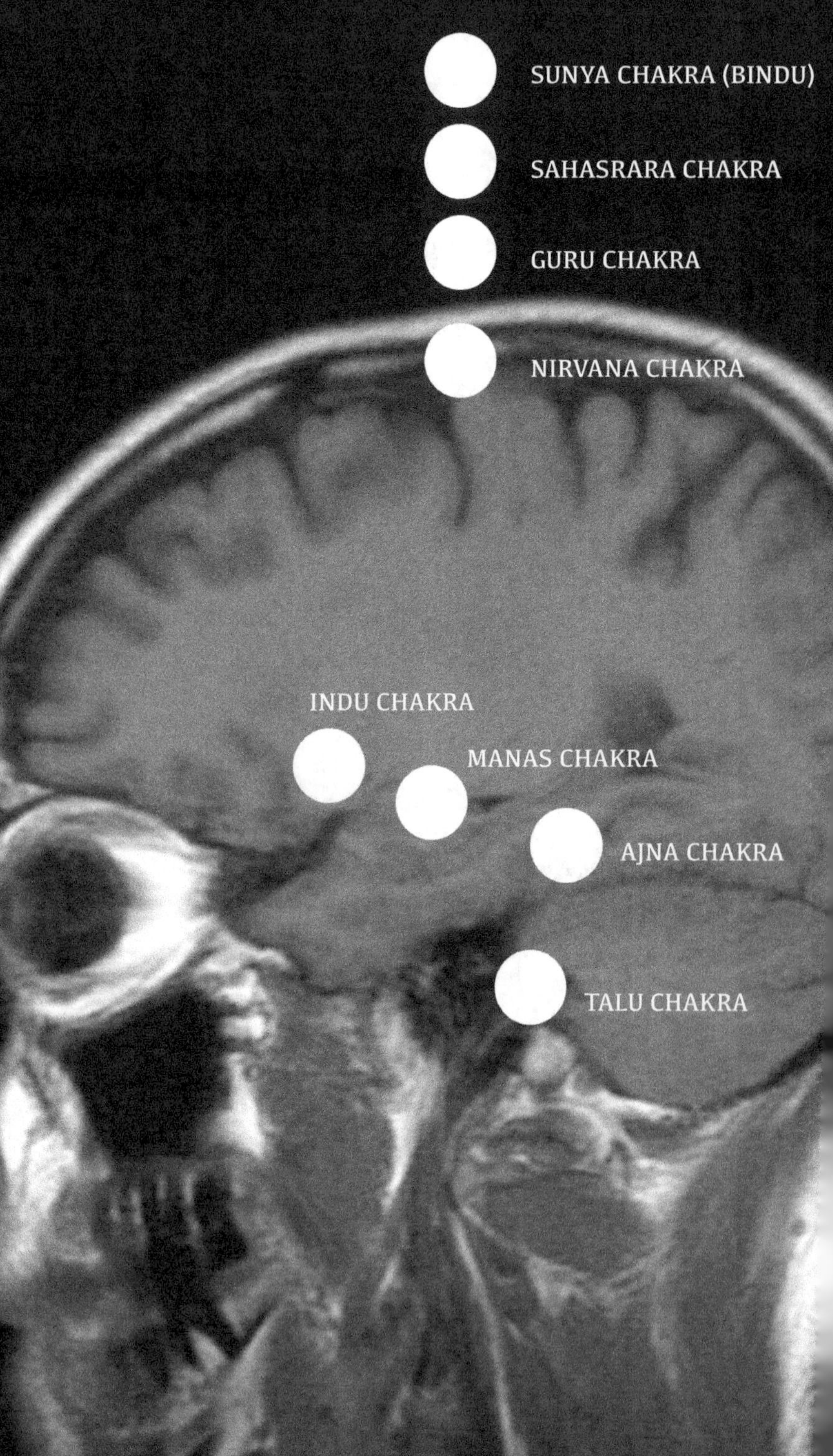

SUNYA CHAKRA (BINDU)
SAHASRARA CHAKRA
GURU CHAKRA
NIRVANA CHAKRA
INDU CHAKRA
MANAS CHAKRA
AJNA CHAKRA
TALU CHAKRA

THE HIDDEN RITUALS

KRIYA YOGA

There are a total of seventy-two kriyas, of which twenty are the most used and are suitable for daily use by any student. These kriyas are divided into three groups:

1. Those who evoke pratyahara.
2. Those who evoke dharana.
3. Those that induce dhyana.

KRIYAS FOR PRATYAHARA:

VIPAREETA KARANI MUDRA

Come into vipareeta karani asana. Make sure that the legs are straight and that the chin does not touch the chest. Close your eyes and breathe ujjayi pranayama. Experience in an inhalation how the amrit or nectar flows along the spine from the Manipura to the Vishuddhi chakra and gathers there. Hold your breath for a while and experience how the nectar gets cool. Then exhale with ujjayi breathing and experience how the nectar flows from Vishuddhi through Ajna, Bindu and to Sahasrara. After exhaling, take the consciousness to Manipura again and repeat the kriya a total of twenty-one times.

CHAKRA ANUSANDHANA

Sit in a meditation position and close your eyes. Breathe normally. Take consciousness to the Mooladhara chakra and follow the front passage "arohan" all the way up to the Bindu. Silently repeat all the chakras on the way up: Mooladhara, Swadhisthana, Manipura, Anahata, Vishuddhi and go from here directly to Bindu. Then let the consciousness go down along the back passage and repeat the chakras on the way down. Starting from Ajna, Vishuddhi, Anahata, Manipura, Swadhisthana and finally Mooladhara. Then start immediately on the next round starting with Swadhisthana. Do not overdo it by trying to locate the chakras but flow past them easily. Practice nine rounds.

NADA SANCHALANA

Sit in a meditation position. Exhale completely. Open your eyes and bend your head down without pressing your chin against your chest. Take consciousness to the Mooladhara chakra. Silently repeat "Mooladhara, Moo-ladhara, Mooladhara". Inhale and let the consciousness flow through the anterior passage "arohan" up to Bindu. Repeat the names of the chakras on the way up. When passing from Vishuddhi to Bindu, tilt your head slightly backwards. Hold your breath and say "Bindu, Bindu, Bindu", silently to yourself. Then continue down the back passage "awarohan" while saying the mantra Om inwardly. Close your eyes as you go down and experience the chakras. When you arrive at Mooladhara, hold your breath and repeat "Mooladhara" three times. Then continue directly to the next round. Practice thirteen rounds.

PAWAN SANCHALANA

Sit in a meditation position and close your eyes. Practice khechari mudra and ujjayi pranayama. Exhale completely and tilt your head down as in the previous kriya. Become aware of the Mooladhara chakra and silently repeat "Mooladhara, Mooladhara, Mooladhara". Then inwardly say "arohan" and inhale with ujjayi breathing along the front passage while experiencing the chakras and mentally repeating their names. When you pass from Vishuddhi to Bindu, tilt your head back and silently repeat "Bindu, Bindu, Bindu". Then inwardly say "awarohan" and exhale along the back passage with ujjayi breathing. Repeat the name of the chakras silently and close your eyes slowly as you move down . Then open your eyes, tilt your head down and start the next round. Practice forty-nine rounds.

SHABA SANCHALANA

Sit in a meditation position. Practice khechari mudra and ujjayi pranayama. Exhale completely and open your eyes. Bend your head forward and pay attention to the Mooladhara chakra for a few seconds. Inhale with ujjayi breathing and ascend along the anterior passage. Experience what the sound of breathing So sounds like on the way up. Experience each kshetram at the same time without any mental repetition. Tilt your head back at the transition from Vishuddhi to Bindu. Hold your breath and experience bindu for a few seconds. Exhale, close your eyes and hear the sound of the breath, Ham. Experience each chakra on the way down without rehearsing mentally. When you get to Mooladhara, open your eyes and bend your head and start the next round. Practice fifty-nine rounds.

MAHA MUDRA

Sit in siddhasana or siddha yoni asana with your heel pressed against the mooladhara. Practice khechari mudra, exhale completely and tilt your head forward. Keep your eyes open at first. Silently repeat "Mooladhara, Mooladhara, Mooladhara". Climb upwards along the "arohan" with an ujjayi inhalation. Experience each kshetram on the way up. Raise your head as you pass from Vishuddhi to Bindu. At Bindu, repeat "Bindu, Bindu, Bindu", internally. Practice moola bandha and shambhavi mudra while holding your breath. Repeat mentally "shambhavi, kechari, mool". When you say "shambhavi", focus your attention on the eyebrow center. When you say "kechari", focus your attention on the tongue and palate. When you say "mool", focus your attention on the Mooladhara chakra. Repeat this procedure three times, accustomed practitioners repeat twelve times. Then first release the shambhavi mudra and after that the moola bandha. Become aware of bindu and walk down the back passage with ujjayi breathing to the mooladhara chakra. Experience each chakra on the way down. With Mooladhara, tilt your head forward and open your eyes. Repeat "Mooladhara, Mooladhara, Mooladhara" and continue on to the next round. Practice twelve rounds and finish with "Mooladhara, Mooladhara, Mooladhara".

MAHA BHEDA MUDRA

Sit as in the previous exercise. Practice khechari mudra and exhale completely. Keep your eyes open. Mentally repeat "Mooladhara, Mooladhara, Mooladhara". Inhale with ujjayi and ascend along the anterior passage to Bindu. As you pass from Vishuddhi to Bindu, lift your head. Repeat mentally "Bindu, Bindu, Bindu". Go down the back passage to the Mooladhara with ujjayi breathing and close your eyes. Experience the chakras on the way down. Then practice jalandhara bandha while holding your breath. Practice nasikagra drishti, uddiyana bandha and moola bandha. Mentally repeat "nasikagra, uddiyana, mool" and experience its seats in the body. Repeat the procedure three times as a beginner and twelve times when you are more accustomed. Release nasikagra drishti, moola bandha, uddiyana bandha and jalandhara bandha. Hold your head down and experience mooladhara. Repeat "Mooladhara, Mooladhara, Mooladhara", mentally. Continue on to the next round. Practice twelve rounds.

MANDUKI MUDRA

Sit in bhadrasana. Keep your eyes open. The body surface under the Mooladhara should be in contact with the floor. Place a pillow or blanket under you if necessary. Place your hands on your knees and practice nasikagra drishti. Become aware of the natural breath that flows through your nostrils. On inhalation, respiration flows through both nostrils and meets at the eyebrow center. On exhalation, the flow separates at the eyebrow center and flows out through the nostrils. Experience how the flow of breathing follows a v-shaped pattern. Be aware of all odors. The point of the kriyan is to experience the smell of the astral body which is the smell of sandalwood. If your eyes get tired, close them for a while. Do the exercise until it feels intoxicating. Do not get caught in it but quit before you are absorbed by it too much.

TADAN KRIYA

Sit in padmasana with your eyes open. Place your hands

next to your body on the floor with your fingers pointing forward. Tilt your head back and practice shambhavi mudra. Inhale through the mouth with ujjayi breathing. When you inhale, experience how the breathing sinks downwards as through a tube that goes between the mouth and the Mooladhara chakra. Hold your breath, experience the Mooladhara chakra and practice the moola bandha. Using your hands, lift your body off the floor and lower it so that the Mooladhara lightly hits the floor. Repeat three to eleven times. Then exhale through the nose with ujjayi breathing. Practice seven times.

KRIYAS FOR DHARANA:

NAUMUKI MUDRA

Sit in a meditation position. Keep your eyes closed throughout the exercise. Make sure to have a pressure at Mooladhara, use a pillow or blanket if necessary.

Make the khechari mudra and bend your head gently downwards. Mentally repeat "Mooladhara, Mooladhara, Mooladhara". Inhale through the anterior passage to the Bindu. Raise your head as you pass from Vishuddhi to Bindu. Practice shanmuki mudra. Block the ears with the thumbs, the eyes with the index fingers, the nostrils with the middle fingers, the upper lip with the ring fingers and the lower lip with the little fingers. Practice moola bandha and varjoli/sahajoli mudra. Experience the passage along the spine to Bindu. Visualize a trident in copper at the bottom of the Mooladhara. The shaft runs along the spine and the prongs point upwards from Vishuddhi. The trident rises spontaneously a number of times and its middle prong pierces Bindu. When it pierces Bindu, you mentally say "bindu bhedan". After a while, release the varjoli/sahajoli mudra, moola bandha and drop your hands on your knees. Exhale from the bindu with ujjayi breathing along the posterior passage and down to the Mooladhara. Say "Mooladhara, Mooladhara, Mooladhara", mentally. Repeat the exercise. Practice five rounds and finish by exhaling.

SHAKTI CHALINI

Sit in a meditation position. Keep your eyes closed throughout the exercise. Practice khechari mudra. Exhale completely, tilt your head forward and experience Mooladhara. Mentally repeat "Mooladhara, Mooladhara, Mooladhara", and then ascend along the front passage to Bindu with ujjayi breathing. Lift your head when you reach Bindu. Hold your breath and practice shanmukhi mudra. Let the consciousness flow continuously down the back passage and up along the front passage while holding your breath. Visualize a narrow green snake moving along the psychic passage. Its head is at Bindu and it bites its tail. When you follow the snake, you can see how it starts to move along the passage or even make its own passages. Look at the snake no matter what it does. When you need to exhale, release your hands and experience Bindu. Go down the back passage with ujjayi pranayama. Repeat "Mooladhara, Mooladhara, Mooladhara", and ascend again along the front passage. Practice five times without interruption.

SHAMBHAVI

Sit in a meditation position. Close your eyes and practice khechari mudra. Visualize a lotus flower with a long green stalk extending downwards. The roots are white or transparent green. The roots spread outwards from the Mooladhara chakra. The lotus flower is at the Sahasrara chakra and is closed like a bud. At the bottom of the bud are some light green leaves. The fallen petals of the flower are pink with fine red veins. Try to see the lotus clearly. You visualize it in chidakasha and feel it all over your body. Exhale and take consciousness to the root of the mooladhara chakra. Inhale with ujjayi breathing and let your consciousness rise along the stem that rises upwards along the spine. At the end of inhalation you reach the bud of the flower. Keep your attention on the Sahasrara and hold your breath. You are inside the lotus flower but you can also see it from the outside. It begins to unfold slowly. When the flower opens, you can see its yellow pollen sprinkled in the middle. The lotus closes

*and opens almost immediately again. When the lotus
has stopped opening and closing, exhale with ujjayi and
go down the stem to the Mooladhara. Stay there for a
while and experience how the roots spread in different
directions. Repeat the exercise eleven times.*

AMRIT PAN

*Sit in a meditation position. Keep one eye closed and
practice khechari mudra. Take consciousness to the
Manipura chakra. A warm sweet liquid is stored there.
Exhale completely with ujjayi while taking a quantity
of fluid to the Vishuddhi chakra along the spine. Stay
at Vishuddhi for a while. The liquid that you took with
you from Manipura is now cooled down. With ujjayi
breathing you exhale up to the Lalana chakra. Inflate
the cold fluid up to the Lalana chakra using the breath.
Take consciousness to the Manipura chakra again.
Repeat the exercise nine times.*

CHAKRA BHEDAN

*Sit in a meditation position. Keep your eyes closed
throughout the exercise. Practice khechari mudra
and ujjayi pranayama. Breathe without interruption between inhaling and exhaling. Exhale and take
consciousness to the Swadhisthana chakra. Inhale and
take consciousness to the Mooladhara chakra and then
up along the anterior passage. At Vishuddhi kshetram,*

*breathing will end and you will start exhaling immedia-
tely. Exhale from Vishuddhi kshetram to bindu and then
down the spine from ajna to Swadhisthana chakra. This
is a complete round. Practice fifty-nine rounds. If you
become too introverted, finish the exercise and move on
to the next kriya.*

SUSHUMNA DARSHAN

*Sit in a meditation position, close your eyes and bre-
athe normally. Take consciousness to the Mooladhara
chakra. Imagine a pencil with which you draw a square
at the Mooladhara chakra. Draw an inverted triangle
inside the square. Then make a circle that touches each
corner of the square. Make four petals on each side of
the square. Take consciousness to Swadhisthana. Draw
a circle there, as big as the previous one. Draw six petals
around the circle and a crescent moon inside it. Take
consciousness to Manipura. Draw a circle and draw an
inverted triangle inside it. In the middle of it you draw
a fireball. Make ten petals around the circle. Take consciousness to the Anahata. Draw two triangles that lie
on top of each other, one with the tip up, the other with
the tip down. Draw a circle around these with twelve
petals. Then take consciousness to Vishuddhi. Draw a
circle with a smaller circle inside like a drop of nectar.
Make sixteen petals around the circle. Take consciousness to the eye. Draw a circle with the sign Om inside.*

Draw two large petals around the circle, one on the right side and one on the left side. For Bindu, draw a crescent moon with a very small circle above it. At Sahasrara, make a circle with a triangle with the tip facing up. There are a thousand petals around the circle. Try to see all the chakras in their respective places. It can be difficult to see everythingat once, start by seeing two at a time and add a new one for each day.

PRANA AHUTI

Sit in a meditation position. Close your eyes and breathe normally. Experience a light pressure on the top of the head, the pressure of a divine hand. The hand provides the body and mind with prana flowing down from the Sahasrara alongthe spine. You may experience this as cold, heat, electricity, or as a stream of liquid or wind. When the prana has reached the Mooladhara chakra, you go directly to the next kriya.

UTTHAN

Sit in a meditation position. Close your eyes and breathe normally. Take consciousness to the Mooladhara chakra. Try to visualize it as detailed as you can. Ssee a black shiva lingam. The bottom of the lingam is cut away and a small red snake moves around it. The snake tries to entangle itself so it can rise up along the sushumna. While it struggles to get rid of it, it makes an angry hissing sound. The tail is attached to the shiva lingam but the body and head rise up along the spine and then come down again. You may experience this as the body contracting followed by a feeling of happiness and bliss. When this occurs, move on to the next kriya.

SWAROOPA DARSHAN

Sit in a meditation position and keep your eyes closed. Become aware of your physical body. Your body is completely still. You are as solid as a mountain. Become aware of your natural breathing while making sure your body is completely still. Your body solidifies and becomes immobile. After a while, you are absorbed by the natural breath while your body continues to solidify. When your body is so still that you cannot move it even though you want to, you move on to the next kriya.

LINGA SANCHALANA

Sit completely still with your eyes closed. Your breathing has automatically switched to ujjayi breathing and you are practicing khechari mudra. Be fully aware of your breathing. With each inhalation the body expands and with each exhalation it contracts. Your physical body is still completely still; it's your astral body that moves. After a while, you only experience the astral body. You may reach a stage where the astral body during contraction becomes a small point of light. When this happens, you go straight to the next kriya.

KRIYA FOR DHYANA:

DHYANA

You have experienced your astral body as a small point of light. Take a closer look at the bright spot and how it takes the shape of a golden egg. When you look at the egg, it begins to expand. As it gets bigger, it starts to get the same shape as your astral and physical body. This form is neither material or subtlein any way: it is the form of pure light.

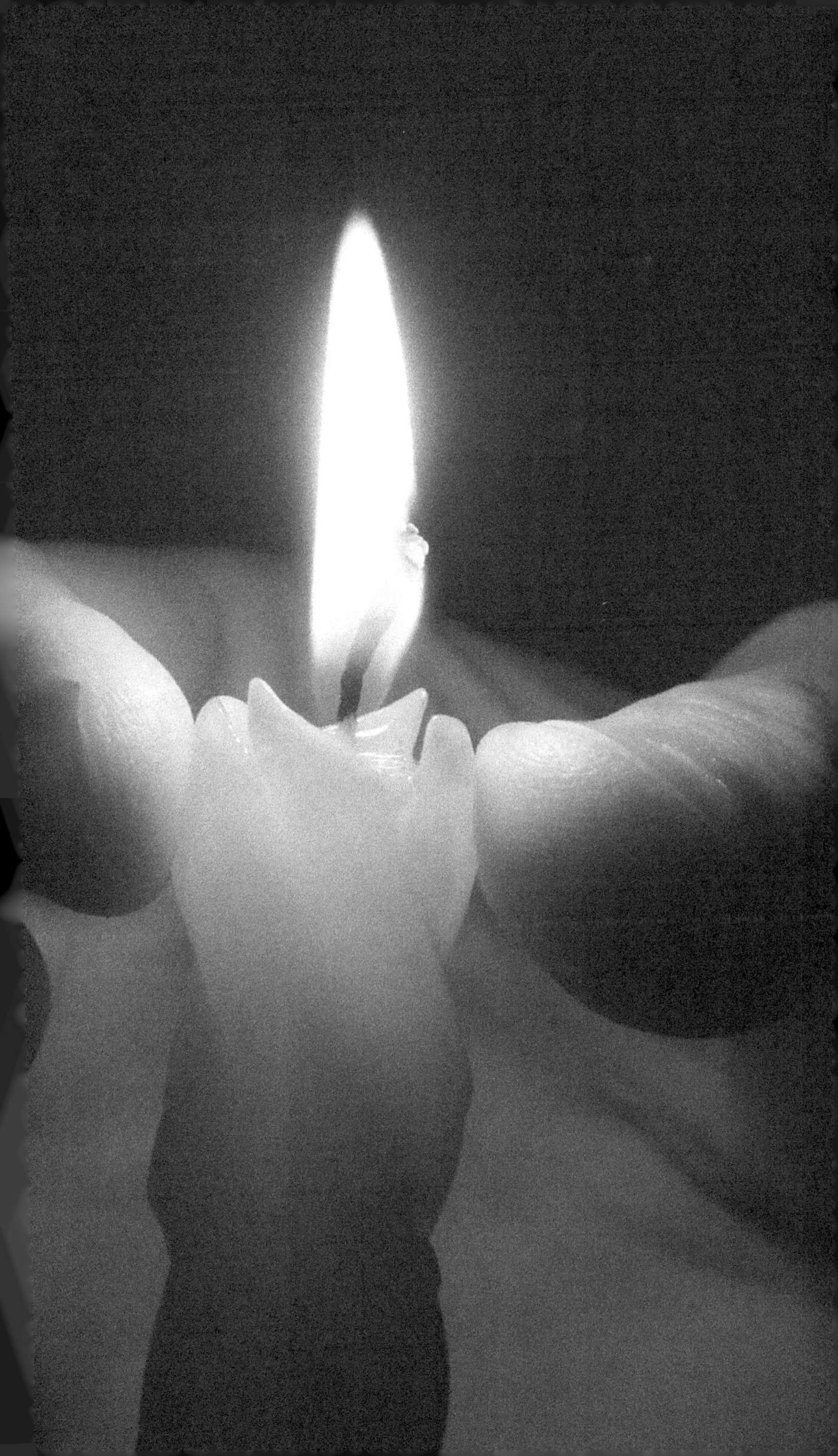

MAITHUNA:

PREPARATION

Everything that precedes the act itself is apt to raise awareness and remove tensions.

1. The room where the ritual is to take place is clean, incense should burn there. The nose and the olfactory organs are connected by nerves and fine psychic currents to the Mooladhara chakra, where the Kundalini is twisted. When the sense of smell is properly affected, your attention and sensitivity increase.

2. Prepare food and flowers to be used during the ritual. The meal consists of four different parts and the room is decorated with flowers.

Pancha makara, tattwa chakra or pancha tattwa is also the name of the five "m" used in the ritual.

Wine – madya.

Wine symbolizes the intoxicating experience of the richness of consciousness, achieved through yoga. If you prefer not to use alcohol, you can replace it with non-alcoholic wine or coconut milk. The element fire. Tattwa agni.

Meat – mamsa.

*Flesh symbolizes, "Everything I am, everything I do
and experience – what I stand for, everything is part of
my being." If you do not eat meat, replace it with garlic,
ginger, sesame seeds, tofu or other soy products. The
element earth. Tattwa prithvi.*

Fish – matsya.

*Fish symbolizes a state where "I experience everything,
the whole universe, pleasure and pain, as myself. I am
all this. I contain all opposites ". If you do not eat fish,
replace it with aubergines and radishes. The element
water. Tattwa apas.*

Roasted barley products – mudra.

*Rice, wheat, etc. They symbolize that, "I stop identifying
with fears and inhibitions". The element air. Tattwa
vayu.*

Flowers (represents intercourse) – maithuna.

*Flowers symbolize intercourse, which in turn symbolizes
the original power, the feminine that rises to the highest
chakra and there unites with the masculine. The element
space. Tattwa akasha.*

3. Swim together. It is relaxing and invigorating and prepares you both to meet your "divine partner". Shakti (the woman who symbolizes all women) is lubricated with fragrant oils and perfumes. Different oils can be rubbed into different parts of the body, such as musk oil around the Venus mountain.

Then you massage your partner's spine in a special way. Start at the lower part of the spine and press your thumbs alternately with small movements back and forth and work your way up along the spine. The area where the sushumna, ida and pingala nadi flow, is then released from tension and activated.

TO OPEN UP

The room has been decorated with flowers, the food has been served and the wine has been poured, incense glows, candles are burning or even better, an oil lamp that emits a red glow.

The next step in this exalted experience is to inaugurate and cleanse the room and the house by sprinkling water and saying a mantra. A mantra with long lines of verse is usually used.

This part of the ritual is extensive and precisely laid out to keep the mind occupied. The mind comes in an

*elevated and secure state. Here you can use the mantra
– Am Hrim Krom Hamsah So-Ham, which is repeated
out loud eleven times. To the house or surroundings,
to the room, to those present, to the food, to the wine,
to the four directions, up and down. The different bija
mantras are often translated as different manifestations
of energy and consciousness. In this context, however,
the mantra as a whole represents "conscious attention".*

*Have a small bowl of water in front of you, dip your
fingers in it and sprinkle the water as above and say the
mantra Swaha (I burn it, I donate it) each time. Also
dip some flowers in the water and throw them on the
food – Swaha, on the wine – Swaha, on those present -
Swaha ...*

*This act should last so long and be so thorough that you
become completely preoccupied with it and can indulge
in it seriously and without reservation.*

*With his finger dipped in red powder mixed with a little
soapy water and oil, Shakti puts a red dot on the eyebrow center of those present. She also gets a point. This
symbolizes the ability for concentration and empathy
achieved through the Ajna chakra in the middle of the
head. If Ajna chakra is aroused, you will participate in
this act without tension, without being hampered by
shame or frivolity.*

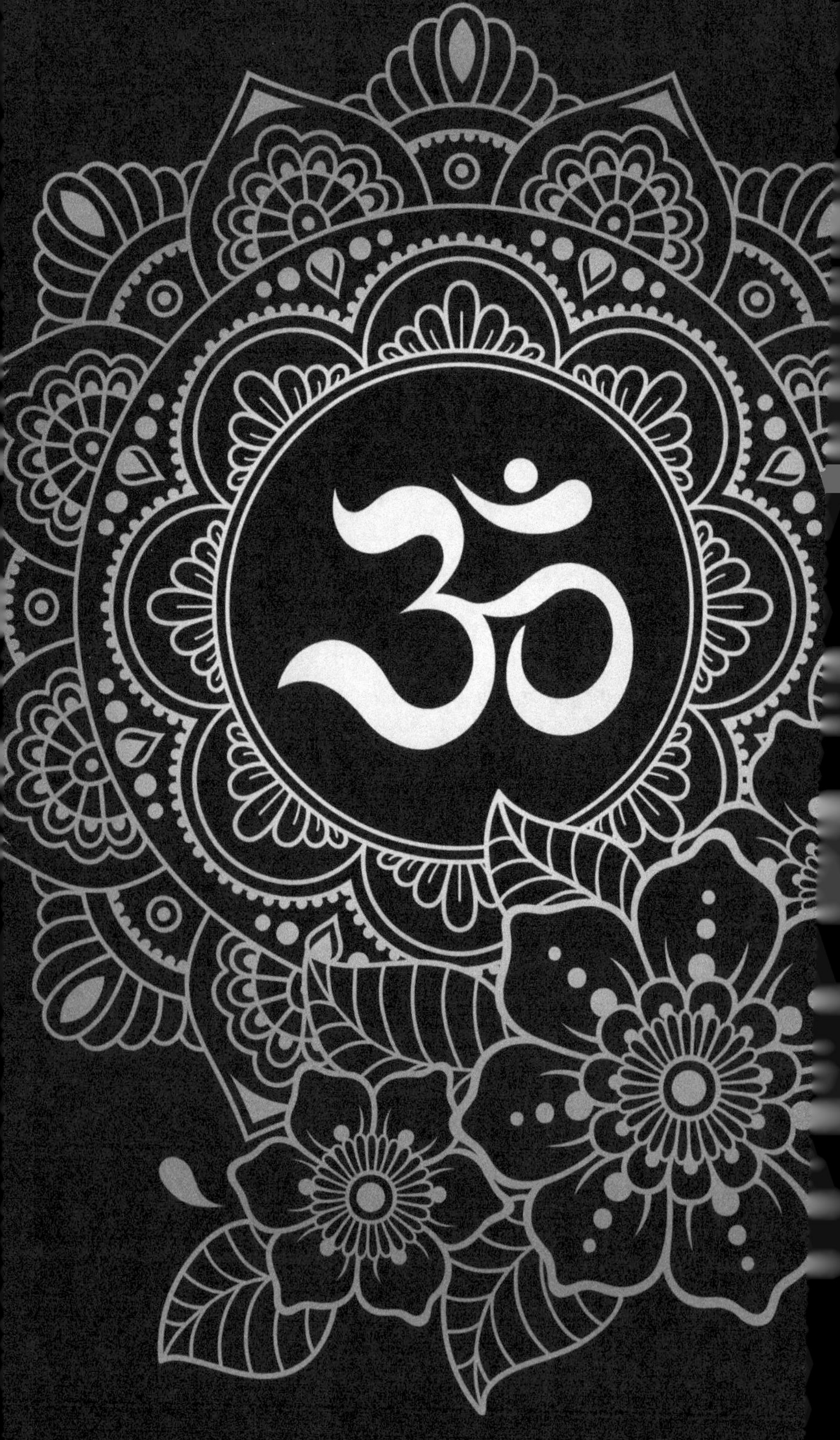

YOGA AND MEDITATION

*Do pranayamas and bhandas and yoga nidra. Then use
the mantra So-Ham (or your personal mantra) with
ujjayi pranayama. Meditate for a while with So-Ham
- So as you inhale, and Ham as you exhale. So-Ham
means "I am that - I am part of the divine, I am God".
Meditate on your body. Experience your natural breathing until you reach a deep and calm state, then repeat
the mental mantra Am Hrim Krom Hamsah So-Ham.
Experience your body as light – imagine that the body is
made of pure light and that this light destroys every fear
in you, every inhibition and all hatred. Experience that
you are prepared for the cosmic act. You experience the
union between the power – the feminine in you, and the
consciousness – the masculine. Experience a strength-
ening and cleansing light flow that fills your entire body
and your breathing.*

RITUALS

*If several people are present, a guru is appointed to lead
the ritual. He dips his middle finger in the water and
draws a downward-pointing triangle on the floor where
you sit and then over this he draws an upward-pointing
triangle. In the middle of both triangles – in the middle
of the hexagonal star, draw a smaller square and in
the square another downward-pointing triangle. A
circle that touches all the corners is drawn around both*

triangles, then eight petals are drawn around the outside of the circle.

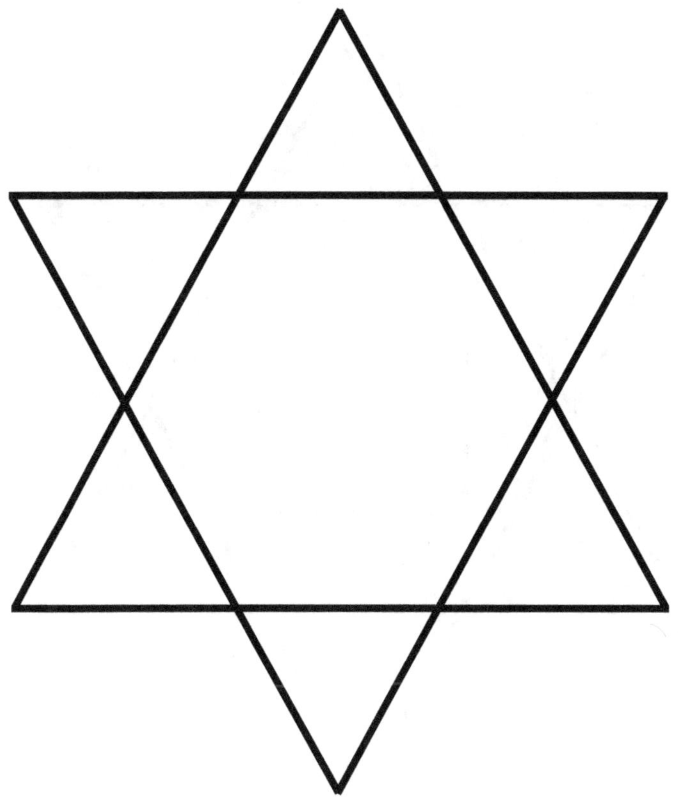

*The two triangles symbolize the female and male parts
of the universe. Shiva and Shakti. Purusha and Prakriti.
Consciousness and energy.*

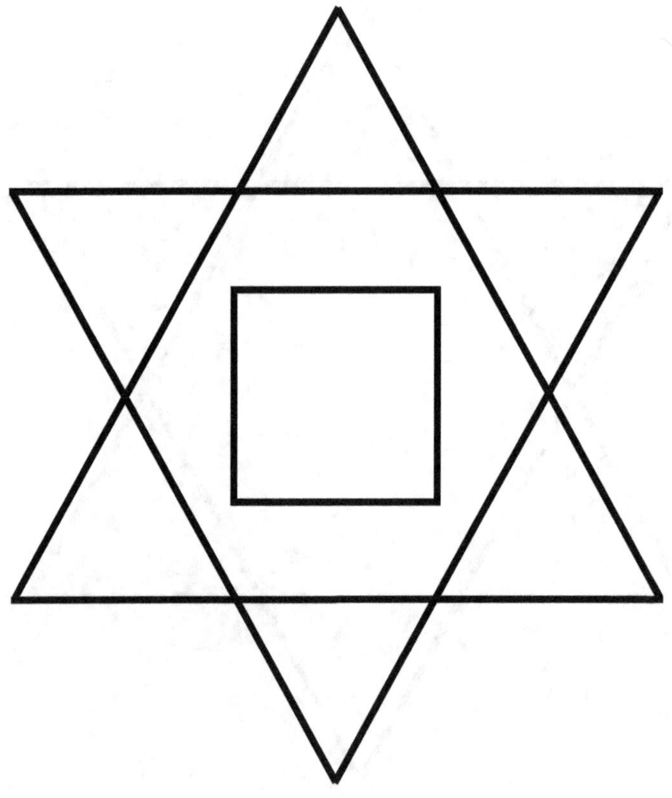

The square symbolizes the foundation from which the power is aroused and rises, the Mooladhara chakra.

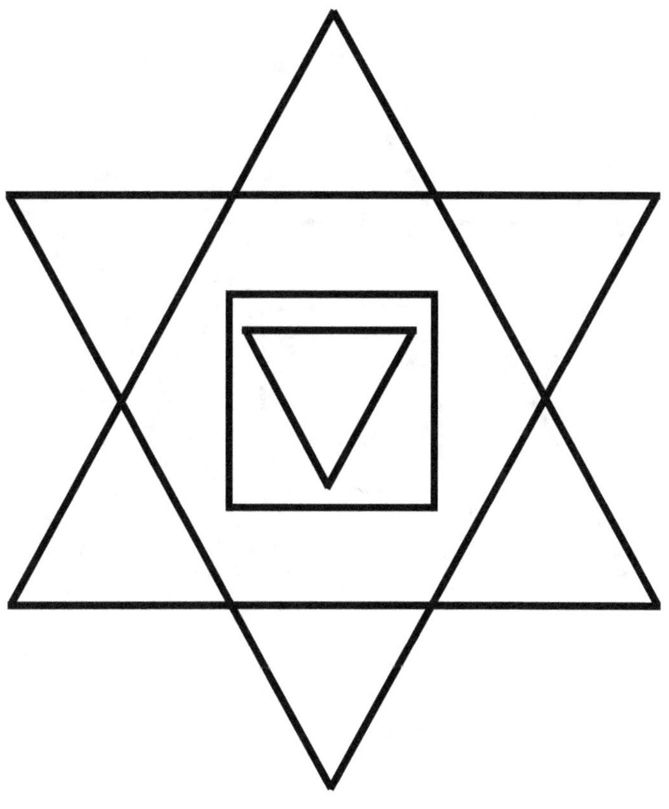

The force, Kundalini, is symbolized by the last triangle.

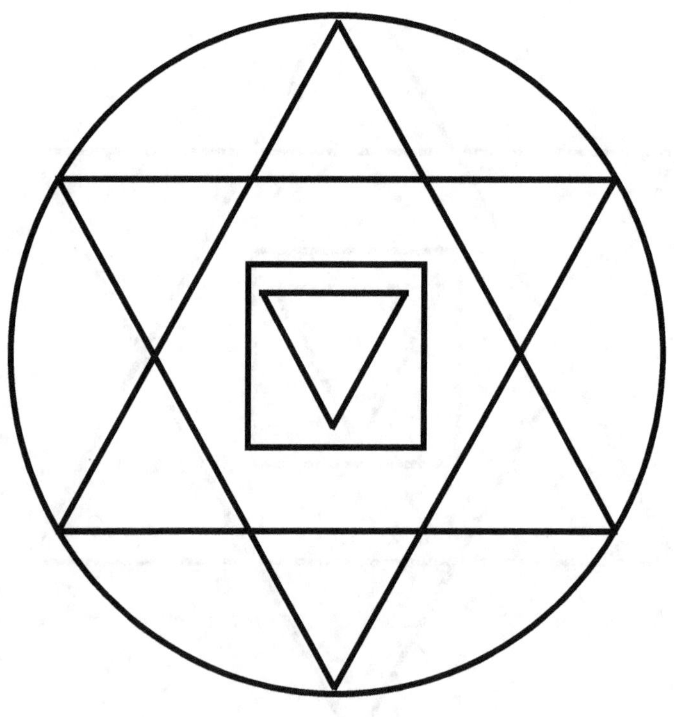

The circle symbolizes eternity.

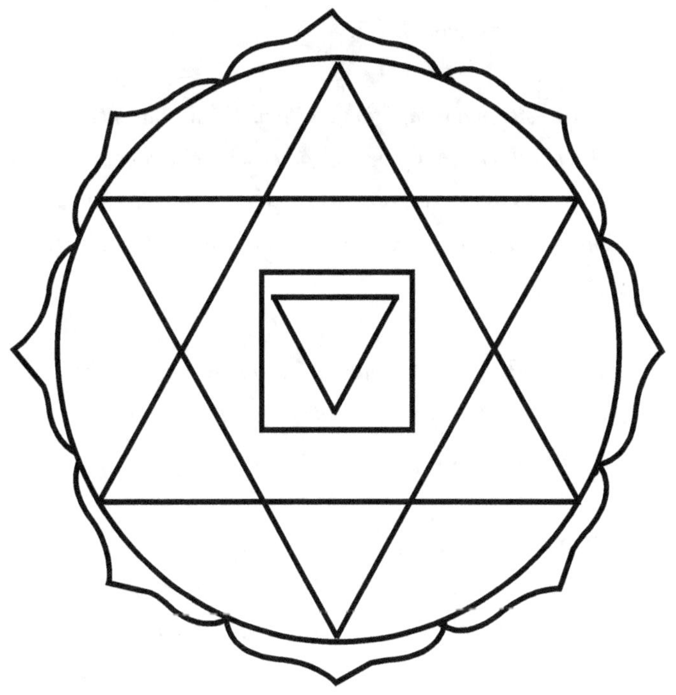

The petals symbolize infinity.

Finally, before the action itself, an important part of the ritual comes: the wine is inaugurated by Shakti with flowers, water and the mantra Swaha. She opens the wine to everyone present. The wine has a liberating effect on the mind, but do not drink too much. Consciousness must pass clearly.

The man sits in a meditation position. The woman sits on his left thigh. They give each other wine and food, feeding each other. If this position too difficult, you can sit next to each other with the woman sitting to the left of the man.

Just as scents affect Mooladhara chakra, Swadhisthana chakra is affected by food and drink. All this increases the desire and sensitivity.

THE ACT

Sit opposite your partner – look each other in the eyes. You are completely naked – two people, man and woman, and experience each other's sex and desire. You appreciate each other; two divine beings, who participate in a universal action.

Meditate on each other, experience each other with desire and joy. If you smile from embarrassment or tense muscles in your face or body, return to the relaxed naturalness every time. Get back to the game and the seriousness of what you do, over and over again. If limiting thoughts arise – whatever happens, accept it and then return to the experience of each other.

Continue to experience your divine partner for a long time. You do not have to demand, explain or excuse anything. You should not achieve anything – just be, experience, enjoy!

The intercourse itself can be performed either in the following way or in one of the sixty-four tantric positions. In the tantric positions you take a sexual yoga position. It is not done mechanically or by you getting up and sitting down again; it is done without you losing touch with each other even for a second. emain immobile in every position...

POSITIONS

1. The man sits in a meditation position and the woman sits down on the man and wraps her legs around the man's waist and hips, so that her feet are crossed behind his seat.

2. Same as 1 – but instead of the woman crossing her legs behind him, she lifts them, while the man holds his arms under her knees and embraces her around the waist and lower back.

3. The man is lying on his back and the woman is squatting on him.

4. The woman starts by sitting as in 3, then she lies down backwards between the man's legs and stretches her legs along his body.

5. Standing. The man stands on the floor and holds the woman, while she hangs on him with her legs and arms wrapped around him.

6. The woman lies stretched out on top of the man or vice versa. There are several different variations, the back must be straight or in accordance with the yoga position. Remain immobile in the position, while you experience each other mentally and physically, together you go into an uninterrupted sexual meditation. You are immobile. The experience of mental and physical union can come at any time and when it comes, stay in it as long as it is at its peak, then end it.

The shortest time in a position is probably a little more than half an hour to reach any real transformation. However, you do not have to worry about the body or the performance, let the Shakti in your partner lead you and your inspiration. Give and receive. Do not strive for a normal orgasm, but let the experience of each other

*transform you. The sixty-four different positions symbol-
ize freedom from expectations, so each time you can do
things differently. You decide for yourself.*

*Get used to the ritual, do it many times. Gradually you
will master it and get the full benefit of it. When it can
be done effortlessly, it will have a deeper effect.*

*In addition to the ritual performed by a couple, there
are rituals shared by several couples sitting together in
a circle. The introductory part of the ritual is performed
by all couples together. The woman chosen to be Shakti
for all present in the circle symbolizes the power and
is honored to be one. She pours the wine and leads the
serving of the food and thus begins the ritual. A guru
performs the mantra ritual and guides the meditation
and the process. During intercourse itself, in the different
positions, each pair sits separately in a large circle called
the chakra. The feast or ritual that raises consciousness
is called puja - chakra puja.*

*Meditating with others creates a strong force field and
provides support to everyone who participates. There are
different puja: In the bhairavi chakra you have a partner who is appointed in advance. In yogini puja, you
choose freely and independently of the individual.*

A chakra puja can be done in different ways. Having intercourse a ritual is so important that it can have a liberating effect on our lives. It becomes a beautiful and central act in human society.

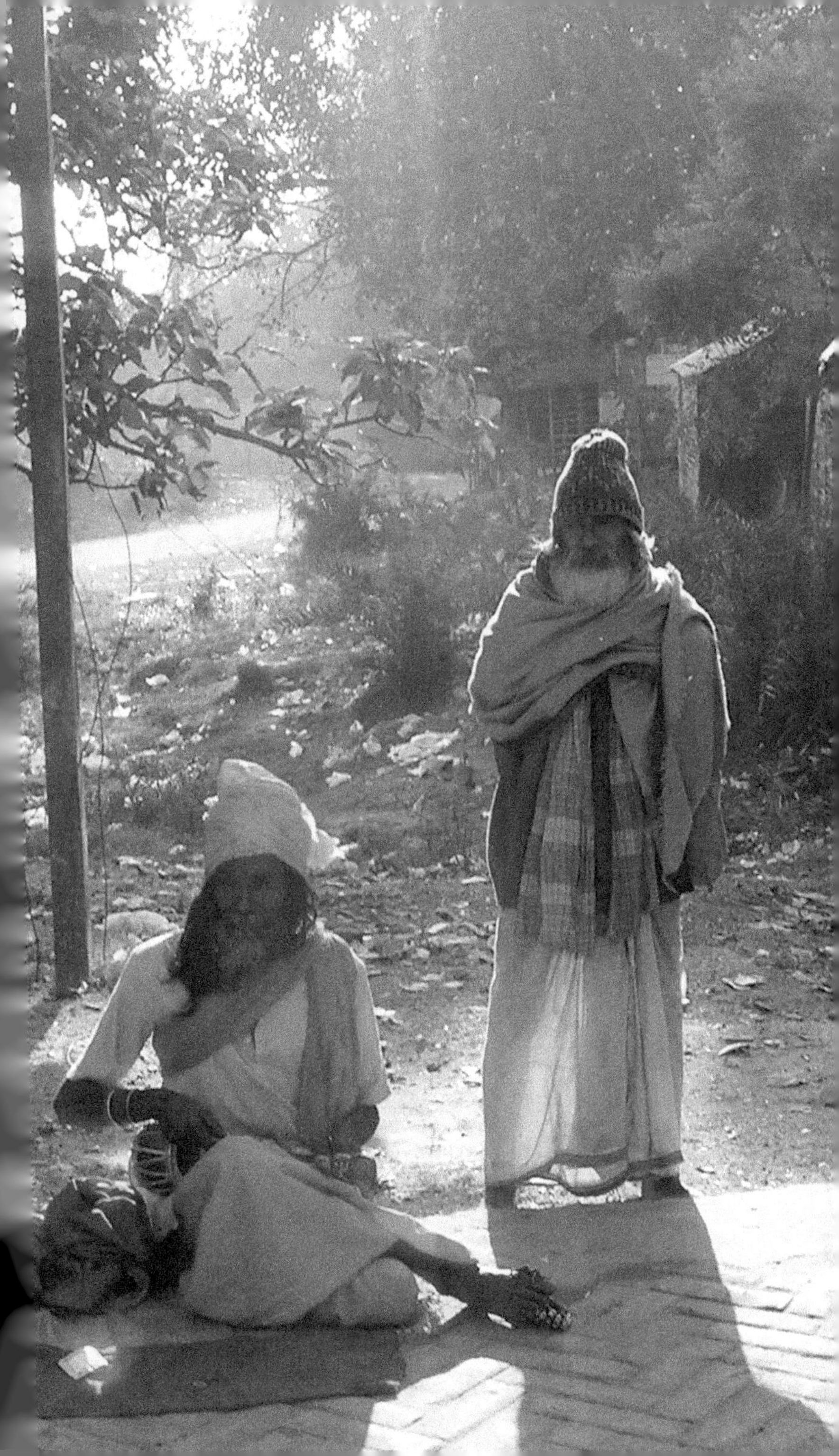

SEXMAGIC

Sexual power and orgasm create life and are the strongest energy in the cosmos. Therefore, it is used in yoga, tantra and magic to give the practitioner the ultimate power. It is quite logical and easy to understand if you think about it.

After initiating sexual magic, you become a magician. The initiation takes place from man to woman and from woman to man. The guru – regardless of gender, passes on his magical powers to the adept via shaktipat. The adept is initiated with the guru's orgasm.

Even if you do not possess the magical power of a magician, you can use your own sexual magic rituals to get what you want, such as, magical desire.

MAGICAL WISH

1. Write down / draw your wish on a piece of paper or use a picture of what you wish. Put it next to you and say the wish out loud to yourself.

2. Start masturbating and experience an inner image of desire in the Mooladhara chakra. Experience how the image is in the chakra and turns dark red in color. Experience four petals that enclose the image.

3. Experience how you draw the image to the
Swadhisthana chakra and how the image turns orange
in color and how six petals enclose it.

4. Experience how you draw the image to the Manipura
chakra and how the image turns yellow in color and
how ten petals enclose it.

5. Experience how you draw the image to the Anahata
chakra and how the image turns blue in color and how
twelve petals enclose it.

6. Experience how you draw the image to the Vishuddhi
chakra and how the image becomes violet in color and
how sixteen petals enclose it.

7. Experience how you draw the image to the ajna
chakra and how the image turns white in color and how
the shape of a pyramid encloses it.

8. Experience how you draw the image to the Sahasrara
chakra and how the image turns purple red in color and
how an infinite number of petals enclose it.

9. When the orgasm comes, you shoot the image out
of the Sahasrara chakra and you mentally experience
how the desire leaves the scalp and goes away into the
cosmos.

Should you change after you have made your magical wish, you will burn up the image of the wish so that it ceases to work.

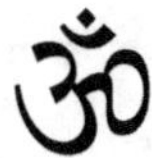